INTERSTITIAL CYSTITIS (IC) COOKBOOK FOR BEGINNERS

Delicious Dishes, Meal Plans, And Nourishing Recipes To Ease Discomfort, Alleviate Pain, Control Inflammation, Restore Balance And Embrace Wellness

DR. JACE ZAYDEN

Table of Contents

Copyright © 2024, Dr. Jace Zayden

All Rights Reserved

No part of this publication may be reproduced, distributed, or transmitted in any form or by any means, including photocopying, recording, or other electronic or mechanical methods, without the prior written permission of the publisher, except in the case of brief quotations embodied in critical reviews and certain other noncommercial uses permitted by copyright law.

DISCLAIMER

The information provided in the book is intended for general informational purposes only. The content of this book should not be considered a substitute for professional medical advice, diagnosis, or treatment.

Readers are advised to consult with a qualified healthcare professional for medical advice tailored to their individual circumstances.

The author has made every effort to ensure that the information in this book is accurate and up-to-date at the time of publication. However, medical knowledge is constantly evolving, and new research may emerge that could impact the information presented. The author disclaims any responsibility for any adverse effects or consequences resulting from the use of the information provided in this book.

References or mentions of individuals, products, websites, organizations, or other names within this book are for informational purposes only and do not constitute an endorsement. The author has no affiliations with, and makes no endorsements of, any third-party entities mentioned. Readers are encouraged to conduct their own research and exercise their judgment when considering any external resources or recommendations.

The author and the publisher shall have neither liability nor responsibility to any person or entity with respect to any loss, damage, or injury caused or alleged to be caused directly or indirectly by the information contained in this book. Any reliance on the information within this book is at the reader's own risk.

By reading this book, the reader acknowledges and agrees to the terms of this disclaimer. If the reader does not agree with these terms, they should not use the information provided in this book.

ABOUT THIS BOOK

This book entitled "Interstitial Cystitis (IC) Cookbook" serves as an indispensable reference for those who are confronted with the difficulties associated with residing with interstitial cystitis. The extensive material is methodically organized to offer a comprehensive strategy for addressing the condition via dietary decisions. By providing a concise synopsis of interstitial cystitis (IC) and its ramifications, the introduction establishes the context for the following chapters.

An important aspect to consider is this book's emphasis on comprehending the dietary implications of interstitial cystitis. This information is vital for individuals who wish to make well-informed decisions regarding the foods they eat. This book explores the practical aspects of developing a supportive diet that is specifically designed for the management of IC, surpassing mere awareness. This resource assists individuals with IC in choosing nutritious foods, with an emphasis on a well-rounded and nutrient-dense approach.

This cookbook is characterized by its comprehensive coverage of IC-friendly recipes for breakfast, lunch, and dinner, in addition to refreshment and dessert suggestions. As a result, it serves as a practical and intuitive guide. It addresses the frequently difficult task of meal planning by providing individuals with interstitial cystitis with strategies that are specifically tailored to their requirements. The inclusion of recommendations for dining out significantly amplifies the practical applicability of this book.

In addition to discussing diet, this book delves into emotional support and lifestyle, recognizing the comprehensive approach to interstitial cystitis management. This book provides an extensive range of practical advice, including strategies for cookery, symptom management, and emotional support, which collectively contribute to its comprehensive content.

Fundamentally, the "Interstitial Cystitis (IC) Cookbook" presents itself as a resourceful instrument that aids those coping with this arduous ailment. Through the integration of pragmatic dietary recommendations, nourishing recipes, and emotional solace, this book provides interstitial cystitis patients with a comprehensive manual for enhancing their quality of life. Concerning interstitial cystitis and the complex intersection of nutrition and health, this resource is positioned to emerge as an essential companion.

CHAPTER ONE

Introduction

Interstitial Cystitis (IC) is a persistent medical condition distinguished by inflammation of the bladder wall; symptoms include urinary urgency, pain, and distress. A critical component of a holistic approach to IC management is dietary modification. The Interstitial Cystitis Cookbook serves as a crucial resource in assisting individuals in making informed decisions regarding their dietary selections, alleviating symptoms, and enhancing general health.

IC can be difficult to manage because symptoms differ from individual to individual and may include discomfort, frequent urination, and pelvic pain. The IC Cookbook is an educational resource that aims to equip individuals with IC with the ability to effectively manage their condition by practicing mindful dining. By gaining knowledge about the effects of food on symptoms of IC, individuals can make well-informed decisions that promote urinary tract health.

An Examination Of Interstitial Cystitis And Its Dietary Implications

IC is a multidimensional condition whose etiology remains elusive, adding to its complex nature. Although symptom alleviation is the primary objective of medications and therapies, dietary modifications can have a substantial influence on both the frequency and intensity of symptoms. By identifying food triggers that may exacerbate symptoms, the IC Cookbook assists readers in adopting a diet that promotes bladder health.

Specific beverages and foods can agitate the bladder membrane, exacerbating symptoms of IC. Acidic foods (e.g., citrus fruits and tomatoes), caffeinated beverages, alcoholic beverages, piquant foods, and artificial sweeteners are typical triggers. Individuals are informed about these triggers through the cookbook, which emphasizes the need for a personalized approach to diet management. Through the comprehension of how particular foods influence their symptoms, people can customize their diets to accommodate their specific requirements.

Developing A Dietary Supportive For IC Management

The fundamental tenets of an IC-friendly diet are predicated on the promotion of bladder health. A diet plan that minimizes irritants and emphasizes soothing, nutritious foods is detailed in the IC Cookbook. Managing IC while consuming a balanced and diverse diet can contribute to one's overall health, and the cookbook provides a road map for achieving this equilibrium.

The cookbook promotes the consumption of anti-inflammatory foods, including hazelnuts, fatty salmon, and flaxseeds, which contain omega-3 fatty acids. Additionally, emphasis is placed on the inclusion of low-acidity fruits and vegetables, including verdant greens, pears, and melons. Furthermore, the cookbook proposes incorporating lean proteins, whole cereals, and dairy alternatives into a balanced diet to promote urinary tract health.

Elements To Incorporate Into An IC-Friendly Diet

The IC Cookbook is an invaluable resource for individuals in search of information regarding bladder-friendly foods that may potentially alleviate symptoms. Even though individual reactions to foods vary, IC-friendly diets can be created by adhering to certain general guidelines.

1. Select fruits and vegetables that have a low acidity level to reduce the likelihood of experiencing irritation. Pears, watermelons, cucumbers, and spinach are some such examples.

2. Lean Proteins: To enhance dietary leanness, include poultry, fish, and turkey in the protein intake. These nourish the body with vital nutrients while preventing diarrhea.

3. Incorporate a variety of foods that are abundant in omega-3 fatty acids, which are renowned for their potential to reduce inflammation. Salmon, flaxseeds, and chia seeds are all fantastic fatty fish options.

4. Opt for whole grains such as quinoa, oatmeal, and brown rice, which are rich in dietary fiber and vital nutrients while avoiding any potential irritation.

5. Dairy alternatives, such as oat milk or almond milk, should be chosen to mitigate the risk of irritation that may be associated with conventional dairy products.

6. Maintenance of proper hydration: Adhere to sufficient water intake to enhance overall health and sustain bladder functionality. Adequate hydration facilitates the elimination of contaminants and decreases the concentration of irritants in the urine.

7. Spices and Herbs: Conduct culinary experiments utilizing spices and herbs such as turmeric, basil, and oregano, which are renowned for their ability to enhance flavor without inducing inflammation.

The inclusion of these foods in meal plans and recipes from the IC Cookbook facilitates the consumption of a varied and gratifying diet while assisting with the management of the condition.

Food Patients With Interstitial Cystitis Should Avoid

Being knowledgeable about which foods and beverages to abstain from is equally crucial as comprehending which to incorporate into an IC-friendly diet. By delineating prevalent triggers that have the potential to worsen symptoms, the IC Cookbook empowers readers to make well-informed decisions and reduce distress.

1. High in acidity, citrus fruits, tomatoes, and their derivatives (such as tomato sauce) have the potential to irritate the membrane of the bladder.

2. Caffeine is present in specific beverages, coffee, tea, and chocolate; it can increase bladder activity and exacerbate symptoms of IC.

3. Alcohol: Beverages containing alcohol may exacerbate inflammation and irritation of the bladder, resulting in increased discomfort.

4. Spicy foods such as chili powder and strong chiles have the potential to induce inflammation and exacerbate symptoms of irritable bowel syndrome (IC).

5. Certain artificial sweeteners, including aspartame and saccharin, may cause bladder irritation and should be avoided.

6. Highly processed and processed foods may contain preservatives and additives that exacerbate symptoms of IC. The consumption of fresh, whole foods is advised.

7. Beverages with Extreme Acidity: Specific carbonated beverages, citrus juices, and energy drinks possess a high acidity level, which necessitates their withdrawal or avoidance.

By utilizing the IC Cookbook as a resource and comprehending the ramifications of these potential triggers, individuals can enhance their ability to navigate their dietary decisions, thereby empowering themselves to proactively control their IC symptoms via dietary means.

To summarise, the Interstitial Cystitis Cookbook serves as a beneficial resource for those aiming to regulate their IC symptoms via dietary means. Through the provision of valuable knowledge regarding the correlation between bladder health and dietary choices, the cookbook enables individuals to enhance their dietary regimen and, consequently, elevate their standard of living. By adhering to a balanced and conscientious dietary regimen, individuals with IC can regain authority over their dietary choices, mitigate the severity of their symptoms, and improve their overall state of being.

CHAPTER TWO

Nutrient-Dense And Well-Balanced Meals

Interstitial Cystitis (IC) is a persistent ailment distinguished by inflammation of the bladder, which results in pain and distress. Management of this condition frequently necessitates dietary modifications for symptom relief. Throughout this expedition, the IC Cookbook proved to be an indispensable asset, providing an assortment of recipes that emphasize equilibrium and ingredients abundant in nutrients.

Consuming well-balanced meals that are abundant in nutrients is of utmost importance for individuals with IC, as they promote holistic health and aid in mitigating potential triggers. The cookbook emphasizes the inclusion of a diverse selection of nutrient-dense foods, including colorful vegetables, lean proteins, and whole cereals. In addition to providing vital vitamins and minerals, these components contribute to a balanced diet.

To ensure well-balanced meals for individuals with IC, it is critical to prioritize anti-inflammatory nutrients. Inflammation-reducing omega-3 fatty acids are present in flaxseeds, hazelnuts, and fish, whereas antioxidants found in fruits and vegetables provide protective qualities. The ingredients in The IC Cookbook have been meticulously chosen to support a harmonious equilibrium between micronutrients and macronutrients, thereby guaranteeing that individuals with IC obtain the necessary nutrients without worsening symptoms.

Additionally, the cookbook emphasizes the importance of hydration for those with IC, as sustaining a healthy fluid balance are critical. Herbal infusions and water-dense fruits and vegetables are frequently incorporated into recipes to promote hydration without causing bladder irritation.

Fundamentally, the Interstitial Cystitis Cookbook functions as an all-encompassing manual, enabling readers to formulate scrumptious dishes that adhere to nutritional tenets and promote holistic well-being.

Breakfast Recipes Compatible With ICS: A Satisfying Beginning To The Day

Breakfast is frequently regarded as the most vital meal of the day, and it can establish the tone for symptom management in individuals with IC. The IC Cookbook provides an assortment of breakfast recipes that emphasize the use of nutrient-dense, bladder-friendly ingredients.

Consistent elements in breakfast recipes suitable for individuals with ICs comprise non-citrus fruits, such as melons and berries, in addition to low-acid fruits like bananas and pears. Oatmeal prepared using water or almond milk, supplemented with grains and seeds, is a widely favored option due to its high fiber and omega-3 fatty acid content. Smoothies comprised of fruits and vegetables that have been approved by the IC are a nourishing and invigorating alternative.

Additionally ubiquitous in the IC Cookbook are egg-based dishes that provide protein without exacerbating symptoms. Paleolithic vegetable omelets or poached eggs with spinach are delectable alternatives that adhere to the dietary guidelines for the management of it.

Through the utilization of an assortment of culinary techniques and ingredients, the breakfast recipes featured in the IC Cookbook guarantee that readers commence their mornings with satiety and nourishment, thereby promoting their general health.

Midday Meals That Are Satisfying And Soothing: IC-Friendly Recipes For Lunch

Lunch provides an occasion to replenish and maintain energy levels for the duration of the day. Individuals with IC must select ingredients that do not induce symptoms of urinary incontinence. This need is met by the lunch recipes in The IC Cookbook, which achieve a balance between flavor and bladder-friendly ingredients.

Salads comprising cucumber, verdant greens, and low-acid vegetables are fundamental components of lunches that are suitable for individuals with IC. For sustenance, proteins such as grilled chicken, poultry, or tofu may be incorporated. The cookbook emphasizes the use of IC-approved ingredients in homemade preparations to improve flavor without jeopardizing urinary tract health.

To maintain ingredient control, the IC Cookbook places significant importance on broths prepared from the ground up, in addition to soups and stews. Carrots, zucchini, and scallions are frequently incorporated into the diet, while common triggers such as tomatoes are avoided. Those in search of a pleasant and calming supper will find convenience and contentment in the following recipes.

In addition to considering potential triggers, the nutrient density of the IC-friendly lunch recipes is prioritized to promote overall health. By being presented with an assortment of choices, individuals can savor flavorful and varied lunches while maintaining their health.

IC-Friendly Dinner Recipes

Dinner is an occasion for individuals with IC to relax and savor a gratifying meal; the IC Cookbook guarantees that this is possible without worsening their symptoms. The dinner recipes emphasize nourishing and flavorful components that enhance overall health.

Numerous dinner recipes that are compatible with IC emphasize grilled or roasted proteins, such as lean meats or fish. These alternatives offer vital amino acids while avoiding the introduction of possible irritants. A variety of roasted or steamed vegetables are frequently served as sides, contributing to the dish's nutritional and aesthetic variety.

Whole grains, including quinoa and brown rice, are often cited as a significant source of satiety-promoting complex carbohydrates. The IC Cookbook offers innovative strategies for integrating these cereals into culinary preparations, guaranteeing a scrumptious and comprehensive evening meal.

Dinner recipes also consider timing and portion sizes, acknowledging that individuals with IC may benefit from consuming a reduced meal closer to nighttime. Through the skillful integration of delectable flavors and conscientious ingredient selections, the dinner recipes suitable for individuals with IC assist in the management of their symptoms while concurrently providing a gratifying evening repast.

Sustenance Suggestions For Interstitial Cystitis: Convenient And Nourishing Alternatives

Individuals with IC may find snacking difficult because many conventional snack foods may contain allergens that induce symptoms. This issue is remedied in The IC Cookbook through the provision of an assortment of nourishing and convenient refreshment suggestions.

Due to their protein and healthy lipids, nuts and seeds are popular options for IC-friendly munchies when consumed in moderation. Incorporating dried fruits such as apricots or blueberries into trail mix results in a gratifying fusion of tastes and textures. Granola bars prepared at home with ingredients approved by the IC provide a portable and convenient option for refreshment while on the move.

Snacks on fresh fruit, specifically low-acid varieties such as honeydew and cantaloupe, can be invigorating. Vegetables accompanied by yogurt-based dressings or hummus offer a crispy and gratifying substitute. The recipes for these dishes are included in the IC Cookbook, which guarantees their adherence to dietary guidelines for the management of IC.

Probiotic-containing yogurt, in particular, is a versatile component of IC-friendly foods. Granola and parfaits comprised of IC-approved fruits provide a delectable and nourishing alternative. Smoothies containing constituents that are friendly to the bladder can also function as a convenient and gratifying midday refreshment.

As a conclusion, the IC Cookbook provides an extensive assortment of refreshment suggestions that accommodate the specific dietary requirements of those with IC. By prioritizing nutrient-dense alternatives and exercising conscientiousness in selecting ingredients, these munchies offer a practical means of managing appetite while actively promoting urinary health.

CHAPTER THREE

Sweet Treats And Desserts Designed With IC In Mind

Interstitial cystitis (IC) is a persistent ailment distinguished by inflammation of the lining of the bladder, which results in manifestations such as pain in the pelvis, frequent urination, and overall discomfort. IC is frequently treated with dietary adjustments intended to alleviate symptoms. Crafting desserts and delectable delights that are compatible with ICs becomes essential for individuals managing this condition.

When developing delicacies for individuals with IC, the principal objective is to exclude trigger ingredients that have the potential to worsen symptoms. Caffeine, acidic fruits, and artificial sweeteners are all prevalent irritants. Conversely, choose alternatives that are more benign to the urinary tract.

An enjoyable alternative is a muffin made with oat flour and banana. Natural flavor is provided by bananas, and oat flour provides a gluten-free substitute. Further, sweeten it with a small amount of honey or maple syrup. Artificial sweeteners should be avoided, as they may irritate the bladder.

Consider consuming a sorbet made with coconut milk for a cooling delight. Coconut milk is an appropriate foundation for delicacies that are suitable for individuals with IC due to its mild acidity. Incorporate natural sweeteners such as Stevia or agave nectar to augment the flavor profile while preventing any potential irritation.

Additionally, anti-inflammatory compounds are advantageous to include. Blueberries and strawberries, among other berries, have anti-inflammatory properties that make them stellar options for delicacies that are suitable for individuals with IC. Generally well-tolerated Greek yogurt accompanied by berries can serve as a delectable and calming dessert alternative.

Replace conventional flour in cookery with substitutes such as almond or coconut flour. These substitutes not only impart a distinctive taste but also aid in the preparation of a confection that is suitable for the bladder. Explore various formulas to identify the optimal combination of flavor and IC compatibility.

Beverages And Drinks

It is of the utmost importance that individuals with interstitial cystitis select the proper beverages. Specific beverages may worsen symptoms, resulting in increased urinary frequency and discomfort. A selection of beverages suitable for individuals with IC is a crucial component in the management of this chronic condition.

Consisting primarily of water is essential for a bladder-friendly diet. Maintaining adequate hydration is critical for individuals with IC, and filtered, purified water is the optimal option. Infuse water with cucumber slices, mint, or a dash of fresh lemon juice to enhance its flavor. Lemon, despite its acidic nature, is frequently tolerated in moderation by certain patients with IC.

Herbal beverages that are calming for those with IC include peppermint and chamomile. The anti-inflammatory properties of these teas may assist in the relief of pain. Coffee and caffeinated beverages should be avoided, as caffeine can irritate the bladder.

Another hydrating beverage that IC patients can generally tolerate is coconut water. Its natural electrolytes render it a more healthful substitute for athletic beverages loaded with sugar. Ensure that the coconut water you select does not contain any artificial additives or sweeteners.

Juices freshly extracted from non-acidic fruits such as watermelon or pear can be a hydrating and flavorful alternative. Nevertheless, exercise moderation, as overindulgence in fruits, even those low in acidity, may induce symptoms in certain individuals.

Avoiding carbonated and caffeinated beverages is of the utmost importance, as they can irritate the bladder. Alcohol should also be avoided or ingested in moderation, as it can exacerbate the symptoms of IC.

Cooking Methods And Suggestions For IC-Compatible Dishes

Enhancing culinary methodologies and integrating targeted recommendations can significantly aid in the preparation of dishes that are suitable for individuals with IC. Individuals diagnosed with Interstitial Cystitis (IC) must refrain from consuming trigger foods and employ bladder-friendly culinary techniques to effectively manage symptoms and uphold a nutritious dietary regimen.

Broiling and grilling are both effective methods for creating dishes that are suitable for individuals with IC. These techniques produce a delectable char without requiring an overabundance of lipids or oils. When accompanied by roasted vegetables, grilled poultry or seafood can be transformed into a delectable and bladder-friendly dish.

An additional method of preparing that is appropriate for IC patients is steaming. The nutrients of steamed vegetables, including zucchini, carrots, and green beans, are preserved without the addition of lipids. Additionally, fish can be prepared using steam to maintain its delicate texture.

When seasoning food, choose herbs and spices that are moderate in nature to avoid irritation. For instance, basil, oregano, and dill are herbs that contribute to the flavor profile without inducing symptoms of urinary distress. Use caution when preparing foods with a piquant component, as they may induce symptoms in certain people.

Incorporate into your recipes anti-inflammatory ingredients such as ginger and turmeric. In addition to augmenting the taste, these substances may also offer potential health advantages for individuals with IC. One potential culinary preparation is a sauce infused with turmeric that can be used with grilled poultry, or a comforting broth that integrates fresh ginger.

Investigate alternative grain options such as quinoa or rice vermicelli, as these foods are frequently more tolerable by individuals with IC in comparison to conventional products derived from wheat. While maintaining flavor, these alternatives provide culinary variety.

Interstitial Cystitis Meal Planning Strategies

Efficient meal planning is a fundamental component in the management of interstitial cystitis. With the assistance of judicious ingredient selection and balanced meal preparation, those with IC can reduce symptoms and sustain a nutritious diet. Personalized nutrition planning strategies for individuals with IC are as follows:

1. Establish a Harmonious Plate: Strive to assemble a plate that is in harmony, incorporating

lean proteins, low-acid vegetables, and non-citrus fruits. To mitigate bladder distress, it is advisable to monitor portion sizes and avoid overloading, as larger meals may contribute to this issue.

2. Conscientious Ingredient Selection: Recognize food triggers and give precedence to alternatives that are amicable to the bladder. Choose vegetables with minimal acid content, such as spinach or cucumber, over acidic foods, such as tomatoes. Select poultry or turkey as proteins, as they are typically well-tolerated.

3. It is crucial to maintain sufficient hydration by consuming water as the main beverage. It is advisable to monitor fluid consumption, particularly if certain beverages have been identified as potential triggers for symptoms. For variety, herbal infusions and coconut water may be included.

4. Meal Frequency: Smaller, more frequent meals should be considered as an alternative to large, intermittent meals throughout the day. This

method can aid in the prevention of bladder overstretching and the more effective management of symptoms.

5. Preparing IC-friendly dishes in quantities and storing them in portions constitutes batch cooking. By doing so, you not only optimize your time management but also guarantee the availability of convenient, pre-prepared alternatives that are by your dietary requirements.

6. Maintain a food journal to record your meals and discern recurring trends in the stimuli that elicit symptoms. This can assist you in making well-informed dietary decisions and modifying your meal plans accordingly.

7. Dietitian Consultation: It is advisable to consult with a registered dietitian who possesses expertise in the management of IC. An expert can offer individualized guidance that assists in navigating food selections and optimizing one's diet to manage symptoms.

8. Incorporate Anti-Inflammatory Foods: Incorporate oily fish, olive oil, and berries, among other foods with anti-inflammatory properties. Additional benefits may be provided by these ingredients in the management of IC symptoms.

9. It is advisable to restrict the intake of processed and packaged foods, as they might comprise additives and preservatives that have the potential to worsen symptoms associated with IC. Fresh, whole ingredients should be the focus of your meal planning.

10. Engaging in mindful dining entails cultivating the ability to fully appreciate each morsel, attentively chew, and be receptive to signals of satiety. This strategy may aid in the prevention of excess and improve digestion.

Through the application of these meal planning strategies, individuals diagnosed with Interstitial Cystitis can adopt a proactive stance in the management of their condition by adopting a personalized and reflective approach to nutrition.

CHAPTER FOUR

Dining Out With Interstitial Cystitis

To effectively manage the symptoms of interstitial cystitis (IC), a chronic bladder condition distinguished by urinary urgency, frequency, and pelvic discomfort, dietary adjustments are frequently necessary. Managing the complexities associated with dining out while having IC can be a daunting task; however, individuals can savor meals without worsening symptoms by exercising mindfulness and strategic preparation. A Cookbook on Interstitial Cystitis is an invaluable resource for developing a diet to accommodate IC requirements. Here are some restaurant dining strategies for individuals with interstitial cystitis.

1. Investigate Restaurants in Advance: Research nearby restaurants that provide options compatible with IC devices before your visit. An increasing number of establishments currently offer comprehensive nutritional details and menus through their websites. To avoid triggering symptoms of IC, choose restaurants that

emphasize whole, unprocessed foods; processed and piquant foods should be avoided. It is advisable to contact the restaurant beforehand to consult about the possibility of substituting or modifying ingredients.

2. Personalize Your Order: Feel free to modify your order to any dietary restrictions you may have. Special requests are typically accommodated at the majority of restaurants. To control portions, for instance, request grilled rather than fried food or request condiments and seasonings on the side. By being assertive regarding your requirements, you can ensure that the preparation of your meal does not worsen symptoms associated with IC.

3. Be Wary of Trigger Foods: Certain beverages and foods have a notorious reputation for inducing symptoms of IC. Caffeine, acidic foods, tomatoes, piquant foods, and artificial sweeteners are typical offenders. Consult the suggestions in the Interstitial Cystitis Cookbook and avoid substances that could potentially irritate the

bladder. Inform the waitstaff of your dietary restrictions, placing particular emphasis on the significance of your distinct requirements.

4. It is imperative to maintain adequate hydration for optimal health, but individuals with IC may experience notable effects on their symptoms due to the selection of beverages. Choose water, herbal beverages, or juices that do not contain citrus. Alcohol and carbonated and caffeinated beverages should be avoided, as they can irritate the bladder. Inform the server of your preference for water without lemon or other citrus slices.

5. Carry Your Dressing: Several commercially available dressings comprise components that may induce symptoms of IC. When dining out, consider bringing along a small container of your preferred IC-friendly vinaigrette. By following this approach, one can improve the taste of their salad while safeguarding their urinary system.

6. When choosing dishes, make an effort to select straightforward preparations. In general, grilled

or roasted alternatives are more bladder-friendly than fried or severely seasoned alternatives. Make a formal request for your meal to be prepared with minimal seasoning or specify which spices should be omitted. Thus, you can savor the dish's flavors without increasing the likelihood of exacerbating symptoms associated with IC.

7. Implementing a portion control system can be beneficial in the management of IC symptoms. To prevent exccss, contemplate ordering canapés or splitting dishes with dining companions. Additionally, smaller servings decrease the probability of ingesting inordinate quantities of trigger foods. It is advisable to scrutinize the portion sizes specified on the menu and inquire whether it is feasible to modify them.

Symptom Management Via Diet And Lifestyle

Interstitial Cystitis (IC) is a chronic condition whose symptom management requires a holistic approach. Dietary choices and lifestyle choices are vital in mitigating symptoms and enhancing general health. Utilizing An Interstitial Cystitis Cookbook as a resource to develop a bladder-healthy diet is highly beneficial. Key lifestyle and nutritional strategies for managing IC symptoms are outlined below.

1. Adopt an IC-Friendly Diet: Managing symptoms requires an IC-friendly diet. Limit or eliminate known triggers, including processed whole foods; these include caffeinated, acidic, tomato-based, and peppery dishes. Meal plans and recipes in An Interstitial Cystitis Cookbook are customized to meet the dietary requirements of those with IC, thereby facilitating adherence to a bladder-friendly regimen.

2. Maintaining adequate hydration is critical for the health of the bladder. Although water is generally considered the most suitable option, certain medicinal teas or non-citrus-based beverages may be tolerated by individuals with IC. Alcohol and caffeinated and carbonated beverages should be avoided, as they can irritate

the bladder. Maintain a steady hydration regimen throughout the day to bolster urinary function.

3. Observe Your Diet: Maintaining a food journal can assist in the identification of particular trigger foods that worsen symptoms associated with IC. Document your daily food intake and any alterations in your symptoms. Adopting a proactive stance enables individuals to identify and exclude problematic foods from their dietary regimen, thereby facilitating improved management of symptoms.

4. Include Bladder-Friendly Foods: Individuals with IC may benefit from the anti-inflammatory and soothing properties of specific foods. Consume foods that are beneficial for the bladder, including vegetables, fruits, lean proteins, whole cereals, and non-citrus fruits. A variety of recipes in An Interstitial Cystitis Cookbook prioritize these ingredients, thereby promoting bladder health as a whole.

5. Stress can worsen symptoms of IC; therefore, stress management is a crucial component of symptom control. Yoga, meditation, and deep breathing are all beneficial practices that can aid in tension relief and relaxation. A cookbook dedicated to interstitial cystitis might encompass details regarding stress-reducing recipes and foods that promote a tranquil and well-rounded way of life.

6. Sustaining a Healthy Weight: Individuals with IC must prioritize healthy weight maintenance. Extra weight can exacerbate symptoms by placing additional pressure on the bladder. To promote weight health, guidance on portion control and nutrient-dense meals can be found in An Interstitial Cystitis Cookbook.

7. Consider Dietary Supplements: Dietary supplements that promote bladder health may be beneficial for some individuals with IC. Glucosamine, quercetin, and omega-3 fatty acids are a few of the dietary supplements that may provide relief from IC symptoms.

Before integrating dietary supplements into your regimen, it is advisable to seek the guidance of a healthcare professional to verify their safety and suitability for your specific requirements.

CHAPTER FIVE

Psychological And Emotional Support For Patients With IC

The experience of living with Interstitial Cystitis (IC) encompasses not solely physical difficulties, but also psychological and emotional dimensions. The contents of An Interstitial Cystitis Cookbook extend beyond dietary recommendations to encompass tactics that promote emotional wellness. Listed below are methods for obtaining psychological and emotional support via an IC Cookbook.

1. An Interstitial Cystitis Cookbook frequently incorporates anecdotes and testimonials from community members who have effectively dealt with the symptoms of interstitial cystitis. Sharing one's personal experiences through reading can foster a sense of community and provide motivation. The knowledge that one is not traversing their journey alone can offer motivation and emotional support.

2. Engaging in mindful dining practices entails maintaining a state of complete presence and concentration while consuming food. There may be suggestions in an Interstitial Cystitis Cookbook for how to integrate mindful dietary practices into your daily life. You can cultivate a positive and mindful relationship with food by relishing every mouthful, attending to signals of hunger and fullness, and valuing the nourishment that your food offers.

3. The mental well-being of an individual living with a chronic condition such as IC may be significantly impacted, necessitating counseling and therapy. Professional counseling or therapy may be recommended in an Interstitial Cystitis Cookbook as a means to confront the emotional difficulties that are inherent in the condition. Disclosing concerns and grievances in a secure environment while receiving coping mechanisms and emotional support are all benefits of consulting a mental health professional.

4. Techniques for Reducing tension: Since tension is a frequent cause of IC symptoms, reducing stress is vital for emotional health. A cookbook on interstitial cystitis might encompass details about stress reduction methodologies, including progressive muscle relaxation, deep breathing exercises, and meditation. Engaging in these practices may facilitate stress management and promote emotional equilibrium.

5. The development of a support network is critical for the maintenance of emotional well-being. A cookbook on interstitial cystitis might inspire readers to establish connections with friends, family, or support groups. Engaging in the exchange of personal narratives, seeking guidance, and gaining empathy from individuals who confront comparable obstacles can foster a feeling of inclusion and provide emotional assistance.

6. Living with interstitial cystitis necessitates adjusting to novel normalcy; therefore, establishing realistic objectives may be

emphasized in an interstitial cystitis cookbook. Recognize and confront your physical and emotional limitations, and establish attainable goals. Acknowledge and celebrate incremental successes while keeping in mind that managing IC is an ongoing process that evolves.

7. Potentially included in Cultivating a Positive Attitude: An Interstitial Cystitis Cookbook are techniques for fostering a positive outlook. One can cultivate a more positive perspective by shifting attention away from constraints and toward the positive aspects of life, including enjoyable activities, cuisines, and daily routines. Positive thinking can assist those with IC in navigating the difficulties of daily life and positively influence emotional health.

In conclusion, individuals afflicted with interstitial cystitis will find the Interstitial Cystitis Cookbook to be an all-encompassing resource. The cookbook covers an extensive range of topics, including emotional support strategies, dining-out recommendations, and nutritional guidance, to assist individuals with this chronic condition in their daily lives. By integrating these practical advice and strategies into their day-to-day routines, people with IC can improve their holistic welfare and more effectively manage the difficulties linked to the condition.

Conclusion

In summary, the Interstitial Cystitis (IC) Cookbook proves to be an invaluable companion and resource for those who are confronted with the difficulties associated with this persistent bladder condition. In its capacity as an exhaustive manual, this publication not only offers a wide selection of recipes but also equips readers with the information necessary to make enlightened dietary decisions that mitigate symptoms and enhance general health.

A holistic approach to managing IC is exemplified by the cookbook's focus on flavorful and nourishing alternatives while avoiding potential trigger foods. This resource addresses a critical void in the existing literature by providing practical solutions for individuals with IC who are afflicted with the frequently incapacitating symptoms of the condition.

Moreover, the cookbook exemplifies the significance of individualized nutrition in the management of persistent health conditions. Individuals traversing the complexities of IC are fostered a sense of community and support by the publication's user-friendly layout and incorporation of expert opinion.

The Interstitial Cystitis Cookbook serves as more than a mere compilation of delectable recipes; it also cultivates a feeling of empowerment by empowering readers to assume authority over their well-being using conscientious and pleasurable dietary practices. Consequently, it serves as an indispensable resource for individuals in search of a comprehensive and proactive strategy to address the difficulties presented by interstitial cystitis.

THE END